Bone Broth Diet Cookbook

45 Healthy and Easy Bone Broth Recipes for Loss Weight. Improve your Health!

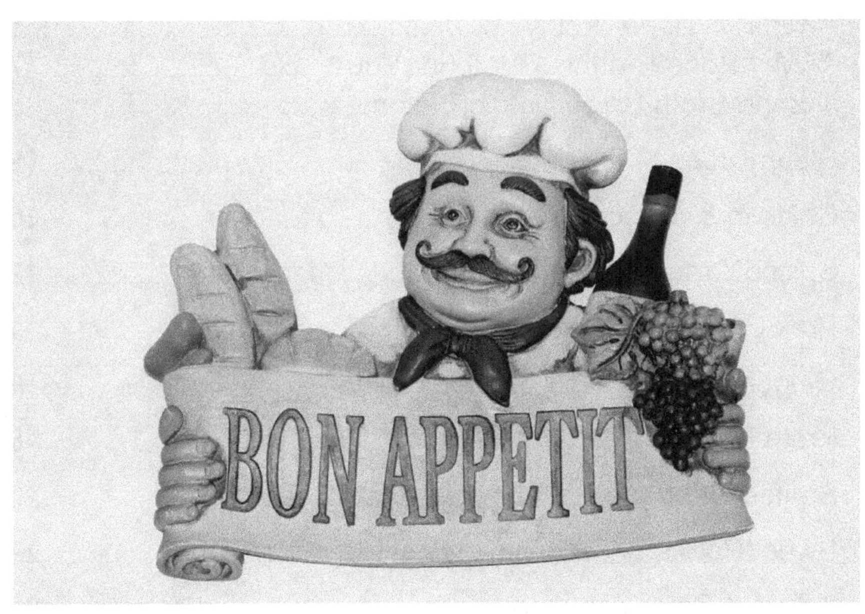

Table of Contents

Introduction

If you've heard about bone broth, you may be asking yourself what this is about. There are many questions that need to be answered. Is it healthy? How long do I need to be on this diet? Have those who used the diet succeeded? I have created this recipe book with 45 different bone broth recipes. When I was doing these recipes, I was aware that for many people, the term bone broth is associated with soup. I can assure you that the recipes I have put together are as diverse as they can come. Yes, there are soups but there are also a lot of other meals you can prepare using bone broth.

Before I look at the 45 recipes we have lined up for I want to discuss the concept of bone broth. The aim is to discuss what this diet is, why it is good for you, its health benefits, how easy it is to use bone broth, and who can follow the diet.

What Is Bone Broth?

It is easy to look at a bone and think that there's no nutrition that you can get from something so dry looking. However, if you look past the hard shell that is bone, there is a hollow part that contains a treasure trove of nutrients. We say treasure because the inner part of the bone has the kind of nutrients that are anti-inflammatory, fats that are healthy, and proteins that heal the gut. This inner part of the bone is where you get the stuff you need to make bone broth.

Bone broth can then be used when you cook other things. The recipe for making bone broth is quite easy. It all starts with you getting some bones. Bones from different parts of the animal will do. You can go for the feet, tails, knuckles, neck or head. If you know how to ask, your butcher could actually give you this stuff for free. Sometimes they actually sell it at a discount as pet food. Put all the bones inside the slow cooker, put the heat on low and allow it to cook for between 6 and 48 hours. What you get on the other side is your broth. You can always include some seasoning or garnishes if you like.

The final product after the long hours of cooking will be clear in color. The color is influenced by the type of bones you use to make the broth. For example, fish bones will produce a translucent broth while your chicken bones will give you a golden hue. Adding other things also influences the final color you get. For example, green vegetables may make your broth take a green color. After the cooking, you can then place your broth in the fridge so that a layer of fat will come to the top of the broth.

You can use the bone broth as a base for stews and soups. This will make your food taste great. You can also buy your bone both from the supermarket but this is not something we recommend. The moment stuff goes onto supermarket shelves there is usually stuff like preservatives added. This can never be good for you if you are looking to eat healthily. Homemade broth will allow you to enjoy all the benefits of bone broth that we have discussed here.

Why Bone Broth Is Good For You

There are a number of reasons why bone broth is good for you. This is the reason why chefs across the world have been using it for many years. One of the reasons why broth is good for the body is that it allows nutrients to be absorbed into the body. Broth provides a source of bio-available nutrients in a way that is easy to digest. This food also comes with a high gelatin content and an amino acid structure that makes it good for repairing the gut. It also helps to get nutrients from other foods to be absorbed more effectively.

If you are looking for a food source that will help your skin, hair, and nails to glow, then bone broth is for you. The reason why it is able to support joint health is that it contains compounds such as chondroitin sulphates and others.

One of the common benefits of bone broth is that it helps you to stay young. It does this by providing the amino acids which help with the production of collagen. Evidence shows that collagen has a way of keeping the skin firm and smooth. This delays the arrival of wrinkles. Other amino acids found in bone broth such as glucosamine, glycine, and glutamine all have an impact on the overall wellness of the body.

Bone Broth Helps Detoxification

During this day and age, we are all finding it difficult to live healthy lives due to busy lifestyles that leaves us with lots of toxins in our bodies. The glycine helps the liver. We all know how important the liver is when it comes to getting rid of the toxins in our bodies.

Now, let's look at the recipes that I have put together. As I indicated earlier in creating the recipes, I tried to make them as varied as possible so that you do not end up just eating the same thing day after day.

Recipe 1

Sloppy Joes

(Ready in 15 minutes with 5 minutes prep time- serves 5)

Ingredients

- 1 tablespoon coconut oil, use tallow or lard

- ½ cup chicken broth, you can also use beef broth

- ½ kg ground beef

- ½ teaspoon sea salt

- ½ cup peered pumpkin, you can also use squash

- 3 tablespoons mustard

- ½ cup tomato sauce

Cooking directions

1. Heat a skillet with coconut oil over medium heat.

2. Cook ground beef in skillet until browned.

3. Add the broth, squash, salt, mustard, and tomato sauce and simmer for 5 minutes until the soup thickens.

4. Serve over a bed of squash, bun, or with tortilla.

Recipe 2

Chicken & Broccoli Casserole

(Ready in 80 minutes with 10 minutes prep time- serves 4)

Ingredients

- ¼cup lard

- ¾ cup bone broth

- 1 small onion

- ½ cup long grain organic rice

- 3 large carrots, chopped

- 2 cups cooked chicken

- 3 stalks celery, chopped

- ¼ kg frozen broccoli, thawed

- 1 teaspoon salt

- 2 cups shredded cheese

- ½ teaspoon pepper

- 2 pints condensed cream of chicken soup

- 2 tablespoons all-purpose seasoning

- 5 cloves minced garlic

Cooking directions

1. In the sauté pan with lard, sauté the carrot, onion, and celery together with the pepper, salt, and seasoning and cook for about 10 minutes.

2. After adding the garlic, cook for another minute.

3. In a large mixing bowl, add the seasoned/cooked veggies and then combine with the rest of the ingredients.

4. Pour the mixture into a buttered baking dish, measuring 9 x 13.

5. Bake, uncovered, for 1 hour at 375 degrees F.

Recipe 3

Spiced Cranberry Pot Roast

(Ready in 130 minutes with 10 minutes preparation time- serves 6)

Ingredients

- 2 tablespoons cooking oil

- 2 cups bone broth

- Salt and pepper

- 2 large garlic cloves, peeled but not chopped

- 2 kg beef arm roast

- 1 3-inch cinnamon stick

- ½ cup white wine

- 1 teaspoon horseradish powder

- 1 cup whole cranberries

- ¼ cup honey

- ½ cup water

- 6 Whole cloves

Cooking directions

1. Use paper towels to pat the meat dry and then add a generous amount of salt and pepper.

2. Use the sauté button on the instant pot to brown the meat for about 10 minutes and then remove and set aside.

3. Into the empty pot, pour the wine, and use a wooden spoon to scrape the brown bits from the pot, leaving it to cook for about 5 minutes. Stir constantly.

4. Add the water, cranberries, whole cloves, cinnamon stick, honey, horseradish powder, and then cook for about 5 minutes watching for the cranberries to start bursting.

5. Put the meat back into the pot, huddling it into the cranberries and then pour in more broth so that the liquid level is almost over the meat.

6. Lock the lid and cook in the instant pot for 75 minutes.

7. Turn the instant pot off, allow the pressure to reduce for 15 minutes and then quick release the remaining pressure.

8. Move the meat to a serving plate and top with some of the cranberry sauce.

Recipe 4

Pork Chops with Leeks and Garlic Sauce

(Ready in 80 minutes with 60 minutes preparation time serves 2)

Ingredients

- 2 bone-in pork chops, make about 1 inch in thickness

- 1 cup chicken broth

- 2 tablespoons dried sage

- 1 medium thinly sliced leek

- 1 teaspoon dried rosemary

- 1 tablespoon cooking fat

- ½ teaspoon salt

- 2 cloves divided garlic

Cooking directions

1. Using a small bowl mix the salt, 1 teaspoon of sage, 1 garlic clove, and rosemary and then use the herb mixture to sprinkle both sides of the pork chops and

leave covered in a refrigerator for 4 hours, overnight is best.

2. 1 hour before cooking, remove the pork chops from the refrigerator.

3. Use a medium skillet to sear chops for 3 minutes on each side before setting aside.

4. After reducing the heat, cook leeks for about 7 minutes watching that they become soft and then add the garlic and continue cooking for 1 more minute, stirring all the time.

5. Add broth and increase heat while the broth comes to a boil.

6. Add the chops back to the pan and reduce heat, allowingthe chops to simmer covered for about 5 minutes.

7. Move the chops to a serving platter and leave to rest while completing the sauce.

8. Add the other teaspoon of sage, and increase the heat while the liquid reduces.

9. Pour the sauce over the chops before serving.

Recipe 5

Ginger Lemongrass Poached Halibut
(Ready 30 in minutes with 10 minutes preparation time- serves 4)

Ingredients

- 4 cups chicken stock

- ¼ cup coconut milk

- 4 cloves minced garlic

- 4 scallions, slice the white and light green parts thinly

- 1 lemongrass stalk, cut into pieces and use the side of a large knife to crush

- ¾ kg halibut fillet, slice into 4 portions of the same size

- 1-inch ginger, peel and finely grate

- 1 tablespoon fish sauce

- 1 tablespoon soy sauce

Cooking directions

1. In a sauté combine the chicken stock, ginger, soy sauce, and fish sauce and then place the fish into the mixture.

2. Heat the sauté pan starting off low on medium heat and bring to simmer before covering.

3. For 15 minutes, poach the fish. Keep checking to make sure that you are not boiling it.

4. Stir in the coconut milk and scallions and allow to simmer for 5 minutes.

5. Test to see if you need any more seasoning

6. Discard the Lemongrass stalks before dividing the broth into serving bowls.

Recipe 6

Broth Burgers

(Ready in 20 minutes with 10 minutes preparation time- serves 4)

Ingredients

- ½ kg ground pork

- Salt and pepper to taste

- ½ teaspoon garlic powder

- Herbs of your choice

- ½ sliced medium onion

- 2 tablespoons cooking oil

- ½ cup beef broth, or chicken broth

- ¼ cup mashed beans

- ¼ cup pureed spinach

- 1 egg

Cooking directions

1. Use a skillet to heat the cooking oil.

2. In a bowl, mix the ground meat, egg, and seasoning.

3. Use the mixture to form 6 burgers.

4. Cook the burgers in a skillet over medium heat for about 5 minutes watching that the burgers brown nicely. At the same time, cook the onions in the pan.

5. Remove burgers from the pan. Keep them covered so that they retain some heat.

6. Add the broth to the pan where you have left the onions.

7. Increase the heat to high and simmer for 3 minutes watching for the broth to reduce and thicken.

8. Serve the sauce on the side of the burgers.

Recipe 7

Stuffed Cabbage

(Ready in 75 minutes with 15 minutes preparation time- serves 4)

Ingredients

- 12 large cabbage leaves

- ¼ cup chopped fresh cilantro, use for garnish

- 1 tablespoon butter, you can use ghee or coconut oil

- 4 cups beef broth

- ½kg beef stew meat

- Fine salt and black pepper to taste

- 2 cinnamon sticks

- 1 medium white onion

For Stuffing

- ½ kg ground beef

- 2 tablespoons ground cinnamon

- ¼ cup chopped fresh parsley

- 2 teaspoons ground cumin

Cooking directions

1. Steam the cabbage leaves until they are soft and place aside.

2. Brown the stew meat for about 5 minutes in a sauté pan with butter.

3. Add the onion, salt, cinnamon sticks, and pepper and allow to cook for another 3 minutes, watching for the onion to become translucent.

4. Use the broth to cover the mixture and bring to boil while covered. Once it boils, remove the lid and let simmer for 30 minutes.

5. While cooking the stew meat, combine the stuffing ingredients in a large bowl and then put ¼ cup of the mixture in at the center of the cabbage leaf. Roll the leaf halfway and then tuck the two sides in before you finish rolling.

6. Add the stuffed leaves into the sauté pan and then cover and allow to simmer for about 20 minutes.

7. Before serving, remove the cinnamon sticks, and use the fresh cilantro as a topping.

Recipe 8

Sweet Potato & Greens Breakfast

(Ready in 22 minutes with 10 minutes preparation time- serves 2)

Ingredients

- 5 strips of bacon

- Salt and Pepper to taste

- ½ chopped medium onion

- 1 box spinach

- 2 cloves minced garlic

- I chopped large sweet potato

Cooking directions

1. Fry the bacon and then set aside.

2. Use a sauté pan to sauté the sweet potato and onion with some salt for about 10 minutes.

3. After adding the garlic, cook for another minute.

4. Add the bacon and spinach and cook until the spinach wilts.

5. Add seasoning according to taste before serving.

Recipe 9

Sweet & Sour Meatballs

(Ready in 35 minutes with 10 minutes preparation time- serves 4)

Ingredients

- ½ kg ground pork

- 1 egg

- Salt and pepper to taste

- ½ teaspoon garlic powder

- 3 tablespoons honey

- Cooking oil or fat of your choice

- 4 tablespoons of tomato ketchup

- 1 cup chicken broth

Cooking directions

1. Mix the seasoning and meat in a bowl and shape into meatballs.

2. In a skillet, heat a few tablespoons of fat and then brown the meatballs.

3. Add ketchup, half of the broth, honey, a tablespoon of fat, and stir while simmering, ensuring that the sauce

reduces and becomes thick. Add the rest of the broth
and continue to reduce. This could take about 25
minutes.

4. Serve with your favorite starch.

Recipe 10

Pork Chops with Pears

(Ready in 22 minutes with 5 minutes preparation time- serves 4)

Ingredients

- 4 pork chops cut into about ½ inch thick each

- ¾ cup pork broth, you can also use chicken

- Salt

- 3 tablespoons apple cider vinegar

- 1 tablespoon cooking oil

- 2 finely chopped Medjool dates with pits removed

- 1 ripe pear

- 1 finely chopped small shallot

Cooking directions

1. Preheat an empty baking tray in the oven at 350 degrees F. while doing the following steps.

2. Sprinkle the pork chops with salt.

3. Heat cooking oil over medium heat in a heavy skillet
    and then sear the pork chops for 4 minutes, watching
    that they are slightly browned on all sides.

4. Move the chops to the baking sheet in the oven and
    cook for 10 minutes while you use the pan to prepare
    the sauce.

5. Reduce the heat, keeping it at medium low and cook
    the shallot for about 2 minutes. After adding the pear
    cook for another 2 minutes watching that it becomes
    slightly soft.

6. Add the vinegar, dates, and broth to the pan and bring
    to a simmer. Cook for about 6 minutes watching that
    the liquid becomes thick.

7. Season with salt and pepper to taste.

8. Take the chops off the oven once they are cooked and
    add them together with any of their juices to the pan
    sauce and combine.

9. Serve pork chops over pears.

Recipe 11

Chicken Pot Pie

(Ready in 65 minutes with 20 minutes preparation time- serves 6)

Ingredients

- ¼ kg boned chicken

- ½ kg frozen mixed vegetables

- 1 can cream of mushroom

- 1 ½ cups chicken broth

For Crust

- 1 cup flour

- 1 cup milk

- 1 ½ teaspoons baking powder

- ½ cup butter

- ¼ teaspoon salt

Cooking directions

1. Mix all the ingredients that are not for the crust and put them in a greased casserole measuring 9 x 13.

2. After melting the butter, mix the crust ingredients into a soapy texture and pour over the chicken.

3. At 375 degrees F. bake for 45 minutes until the crust is golden.

4. Serve.

Recipe 12

Garlic & Ginger Beef

(Ready in 45 minutes with preparation time of 30 minutes- serves 4)

Ingredients

- 5 tablespoon soy sauce (divide)

- 1 head fresh broccoli, cut into florets

- 1 ½ tablespoons sunflower oil (divided)

- ½ kg beef sirloin (cut along the grain into ¼ inch slices)

- 1 teaspoon dried ginger

- 3 tablespoons cooking oil

- 1 teaspoon garlic powder, granulated (divide)

- 1 teaspoon arrowroot powder

- ¼ cup beef broth

- 1 tablespoon sunflower oil

Cooking directions

1. Make the marinade by mixing ½ teaspoon of garlic, fish sauce, 2 tablespoons soy sauce, ginger, and 1 tablespoon sesame oil in a bowl.

2. Put in the beef and allow it to marinate for 30 minutes at room temperature.

3. In the meantime, prepare the sauce by combining the arrowroot powder, 3 tablespoons soy sauce, ½ teaspoon garlic, and ½ teaspoon sunflower oil, and then set aside.

4. Over medium heat in a large skillet, heat 2 tablespoons of coconut oil and then cook the meat in one layer for about 2 minutes. Then turn and cook the other side for another 2 minutes ensuring that the meat browns.

5. Remove the meat and put aside.If there is no more oil in the pan, add one more tablespoon of coconut oil.

6. After adding the broccoli, cook for another minute.

7. Add 2 tablespoons of water and cook covered for 3 minutes then after removing the cover, cook until the broccoli reaches your desired state of doneness.

8. Put the meat back into the pan and add the sauce before combining well.

9. Serve with a topping of your choice.

Recipe 13

Chicken Stroganoff

(Ready in 18 minutes with preparation time of 10 minutes- serves 4)

Ingredients

- ½ground chicken

- ½ teaspoon garlic powder

- 1 tablespoon lard

- ½ teaspoon pepper

- 1 diced small onion

- 1 teaspoon sea salt to taste

- ½ cup chicken broth

- 1 tablespoon tapioca flour

- ½ cup milk

Cooking directions

1. Heat the lard in a large skillet and then brown the meat and onions.

2. Add the seasoning, milk, and broth and allow to simmer for 5 minutes.

3. In 1 tablespoon of cold water, mix in the arrowroot.

4. Add the mixture into the pan and allow to simmer into a
    thick paste; this should take about 3 minutes.

5. After adjusting the seasoning, serve over
    carbohydrates of your choice.

Recipe 14

Wonton Soup

(Ready in 40 minutes with 35 minutes prep time- serves 4)

Ingredients

- 1 wonton filling

- 2 cans (400g each) chicken broth with reduced sodium

- Coarse salt to taste

- 3 thinly sliced scallions

- 3 teaspoons rice vinegar

- ½ teaspoon toasted sesame oil

Cooking directions

1. In a large bowl, make the soup by combining 4 cups of water, the salt, and broth.

2. Bring to boil.

3. The wontons should be added one at a time and allowed to boil again.

4. When all the wontons are in, reduce the heat and cook the wontons slowly until they are cooked. This should take about 6 minutes.

5. Stir in the sesame oil, salt, vinegar, and sesame oil.

6. Serve the soup.

Recipe 15

Chicken & Broccoli Casserole

(Ready in 50 minutes with 10 minutes prep time- serves 4)

Ingredients

- ½ cup olive oil, have some additional olive oil

- 4 slices whole wheat bread

- 3 ½ cups chopped onions

- 220g fresh crab meat

- 2 medium fennel bulbs with fronds, core the bulbs and thinly slice them and chop the fronds and put aside

- 2 cups vegetable broth, you can use more

- 3 minced large garlic cloves

- 2 400ml cans diced tomatoes in juice

Cooking directions

1. In a large, heavy pot, heat a ¼ cup of oil over medium heat.

2. Add the onions garlic, funnel slices, and add some salt and pepper.

3. Sauté the onions until they are tender. This should take about 15 minutes. If the onions brown too rapidly, reduce the heat.

4. Add the broth and onions and allow to boil.

5. Cook for 15 more minutes on reduced heat.

6. Add the crabmeat. If desired add more cups of broth and allow to heat for another 4 minutes or so.

7. Season the soup with salt and pepper.

8. Before serving the soup in bowls, sprinkle the fennels fronds over and drizzle some oil over each serving.

9. Serve with toast.

Recipe 16

Mashed Potatoes

(Ready in 35 minutes with 15 minutes prep time- serves 5)

Ingredients

- 2 cups of chicken broth

- 5 large peeled and cubed Yukon golden potatoes

- ½ cup of organic milk cream

- 2 tablespoons butter

- Salt to taste

Cooking directions

1. Using a 3-quart saucepan bring broth and potatoes to boil over medium-high heat

2. Regulate the heat to medium. Cook until the potatoes are tender, about 10 minutes. Use a colander to drain the potatoes, reserve the broth.

3. Mash the potatoes with cream, reserved broth and butter. Season with salt.

Steamed Vegetables

(Ready in 20 minutes with 10 minutes prep time- serves 4)

Ingredients

- 2 cups of vegetable broth

- 1 cup of cauliflower florets

- 1 cup of broccoli florets

- ½ cup of chopped celery stalks

- ½ cup of peeled and chopped carrots

Cooking directions

1. Bring the vegetables and broth to boil.

2. Reduce the heat to low.

3. Cook until the vegetables are tender, about 5 minutes.

4. Before serving, drain the vegetables.

Recipe 18

Beef Bloody Mary

(Ready in 1 hour 15 minutes with 10 minutes preparation time- serves 4)

Ingredients

- 2 cups of vegetable broth

- 2 tablespoon of fresh orange juice

- 4 sliced cucumber

- 4 twigs of fresh thyme leaves

- ½ teaspoon soy sauce

- 1 teaspoon hot pepper sauce

- ½ teaspoon black pepper

- 2/3 ounces fluid vodka

- 2 teaspoon of Worcestershire sauce

- 1 cup V8 original

Cooking directions

1. In a medium pitcher, mix all the ingredients expect
   thyme and cucumber. Keep in a refrigerator for 1 hour.

2. Fill four glasses with ice. Divide the mixture above into
    the glasses

3. Garnish with the thyme sprigs and cucumber slices.

4. Ready to serve.

Recipe 19

Chicken Dumplings

(Ready in 45 minutes with 15 minutes preparation time serves 4)

Ingredients

- 2 cups chicken broth

- 8 cubed chicken breasts, skinless and boneless

- 1 package baby carrots

- I chopped onion

- 2 sliced celery stalks

- Salt and black pepper to taste

- 2 bay leaves

- 21/4 cups baking mix

- 1 cup of milk

Cooking directions

1. In a large pan, mix onion, carrot, bay leaves, chicken, broth, pepper and salt, and heat to boil. Cover the pot and reduce the heat. Cook until the vegetables are

tender and the chicken loses the pink color, about 25 minutes.

2. In a bowl combine the baking and milk, forming sticky dough. Make golf ball-sized pieces of dough and drop them into the soup. Cook for about 10 minutes, until the dumplings are cooked through.

3. Ready to serve

Recipe 20

Slow Cooker Caveman Chili

(Ready in 4 hrs. 30minutes with 15 minutes preparation time- serves 4)

Ingredients

- 11/2 pounds cubed beef

- 1 package of bacon

- 2 tablespoons of coconut oil

- 1 teaspoon kosher salt

- I medium sized red onion, sliced

- 2 coarsely chopped garlic cloves

- I organic red pepper, cut into small chunks

- 2 celery stalks, chopped

- 2 cups of diced fresh organic tomatoes

- 1 cup of vegetable broth

- 1 tablespoon chili powder

- I teaspoon of turmeric powder

- 1 tablespoon cacao powder

- 2 tablespoons honey

Cooking directions

1. Cook bacon until crispy, about 20 minutes. Set aside.

2. In a large saucepan, melt 1 tablespoon of coconut oil. Add half of the beef, and season it with salt. Cook until it turns brown on all sides, about 5 minutes. Add to the slow cooker.

3. Season the other half of beef like above, and add it to the slow cooker too.

4. Use the same saucepan to melt 2 tablespoon of butter. Sauté onions and garlic and cook until they turn light brown, about 3 minutes. Add the cooked onions to the slow cooker.

5. Add all the other ingredients and stir gently to combine.

6. Cover with a lid and cook on high heat for 4 hours, until the meat is tender.

7. Serve hot with bacon toppings.

Recipe 21

Thai Chicken & Vegetable Soup

(Ready in 45 minutes with 30 minutes preparation time- serves 5)

Ingredients

- ½ cup of carrots sliced into matchstick like stripes

- 1 tablespoon coconut oil

- 11/2 cups red pepper, cubed

- 1 cup sliced mushrooms

- 2 cups chicken broth

- 2 tablespoons of ginger root, peeled and minced

- ¼ teaspoon of cayenne pepper

- 2 tablespoons lemon juice

- 14 ounces (1 can) coconut milk, unsweetened

- 2 cups cubed chicken breast, boneless

- 2 teaspoon grated lime zest

- 11/2 teaspoon lemon zest, grated

- 2 tablespoons fresh cilantro, chopped

Cooking directions

1. Over medium heat put the oil in a 4-quart saucepan. Add pepper and carrot, stir occasionally and cook until tender. Add mushrooms, stir and cook for a minute. Add the cayenne pepper and ginger, stir and cook for 30 seconds.

2. Add coconut milk and broth and bring to boil. Regulate the heat to medium. Cook for about 5 minutes. Add chicken, stir and cook until hot.

3. Remove saucepan from the heat.

4. Add lime zest, lemon zest, and lemon juice, and stir. Add salt to taste.

5. Just before serving, add cilantro.

Recipe 22

Roasted Asparagus Soup

(Ready in 43 minutes with 15 minutes preparation time- serves 6)

Ingredients

- 2 pounds of trimmed asparagus spears

- 6 cups of vegetable broth

- 3 tablespoons coconut oil

- 3 tablespoons of all-purpose flour

- 1 large coarsely chopped sweet onion

- 3 minced gloves of garlic

- ½ cup organic milk cream

Cooking directions

1. Preheat the oven to 425 degrees F.

2. On a rimmed baking sheet, place the asparagus and sprinkle 1 tablespoon oil.

3. Roast the asparagus until tender, about 10 minutes. Leave to cool and chop into small pieces, about 1-inch.

4. While roasting the asparagus, pour the remaining oil in a 4-quart saucepot and heat it over medium heat. Add garlic and onion, cook until the onions are tender, about 5 minutes.

5. Lower the heat. To the onion mixture add flour, and cook for about 5 minutes. Add broth and stir gradually. Bring to boil, and cook for about 10 minutes.

6. Add the roasted asparagus to the saucepan.

7. Blend the mixture until it is smooth.

8. Add organic cream and continue blending, until evenly mixed.

9. Add salt to taste.

10. Ready to serve.

Garlic-Ginger Beef & Noodle Soup

(Ready in 30 minutes with 10 minutes preparation time- serves 4)

Ingredients

- 4 cups of beef broth

- 1 tablespoon olive oil

- 1 pound minced beef top sirloin steak

- ½ cup minced garlic

- 3 teaspoons of fresh ginger, minced

- 4 ounces of thin spaghetti noodles, broken into thirds, uncooked

- 1 package stir-fry vegetable blend, frozen

- 1 tablespoon soy sauce

Cooking directions

1. In a large bowl mix 2 teaspoons ginger, 1 tablespoon garlic, olive oil, and beef; toss to coat. Marinate it in refrigerator while covered, for about 30 minutes to 2 hours.

2. In a large pan combine broth with the remaining ginger, garlic, and heat to boil. Add pasta and vegetables, stir and boil. Reduce the heat. Keep the pan uncovered until the vegetables and pasta are tender, about 6 minutes. Remember to stir occasionally.

3. In the meantime, over a medium-high heat, heat a large nonstick skillet until hot. Add the remaining beef, fry and stir until the pink color disappears. Remove the skillet and repeat the same process on the other half. Set it aside and keep warm.

4. Remove the soup from heat, and add beef. Season with soy sauce.

5. Ready to serve.

Recipe 24

Shepherd's Pie

(Ready in 55 minutes with 10 minutes preparation time- serves 4)

Ingredients

- ¾ cup beef broth

- ¼ cup of shredded Cheddar Cheese

- 2 tablespoons of all-purpose floor

- 1 tablespoon ketchup

- 1 pound lean beef, grounded

- 1 tablespoon olive oil

- 1 chopped onion

- 5 chopped carrots

- 1 tablespoon butter

- Salt and pepper to taste

- 4 large peeled and cubed potatoes

- 1 tablespoon onion, finely chopped

Cooking directions

1. In a large pot boil salted water.

2. Add potatoes for 15 minutes or cook until tender. Drain them. Mash and combine with butter, ¼ cup cheese, and finely chopped onion. Add salt and pepper to taste. Keep aside.

3. Boil salted water on a large pot. Add carrot for about 15 minutes or cook until tender but still firm. Drain the excess water, wash, and keep aside.

4. Preheat oven to 190 degrees C

5. In a large frying pan heat oil. Add chopped onion, cook until clear. Stir ground beef and cook until brown. Drain the excess fat, stir the beef mixture in flour and cook for a minute. Add broth and ketchup. Heat to boil, then regulate heat, and simmer for about 5 minutes.

6. On the bottom of the baking dish spread an even layer of ground beef, add smashed carrots, cover with mashed potatoes, and sprinkle with remaining cheese.

7. Bake until golden brown, for about 20 minutes.

Recipe 25

Melt-in-Your-Mouth Pot Roast

(Ready in 6 hours 10 minutes with 10 minutes preparation time- serves 4)

Ingredients

- 1 cup baby carrots, fresh

- 1 cup beef broth

- 1 pound quartered medium red potatoes

- 4 pounds boneless beef chuck, roasted

- 2 teaspoons of dried and crushed rosemary

- ¼ cup Dijon mustard

- 1-2teaspoons thyme, dried

- 1 teaspoon of garlic salt

- 1/3 cup sliced onions

- ½ teaspoon pepper

Cooking directions

1. In a 5-quart slow cooker place potatoes. Divide the beef roast into two. Rub a mixture of rosemary, mustard, thyme, garlic salt, and pepper over roast.

2. Place the cooker on medium heat, and add onion and broth. Cook until the vegetables and meat are tender, about 6 hours.

3. Sprinkle cooking juices on the mixture, marinated in a freezer, until roast and vegetables cook and freeze.

4. Heat the mixture in a saucepan, stir gently and add some water if need be.

5. Ready to serve.

Vegetable Lo Mein

(Ready in 35 minutes with 10 minutes preparation time- serves 2)

Ingredients

- 1 cup chicken broth

- 8 ounces spaghetti uncooked

- 2 cups mushroom, fresh and sliced

- 1 chopped onion

- 1 cup carrots, shredded

- ¼ cup coconut oil

- 2 cups been sprout, fresh

- 2 minced garlic cloves

- 1 tablespoon of cornstarch

- ½ cup green onion, chopped

- 1 tablespoon soy sauce

- 2 tablespoons of original honey

- ¼ teaspoon of curry powder

- ¼ teaspoon of cayenne

- 1teaspoon fresh ginger, grated

- ¼ cup of hoisin sauce

Cooking directions

1. In a large pot, heat salted water to boil. Add pasta, and cook until tender for about 8-10 minutes. Set aside.

2. In a large saucepan heat oil. Fry carrots, peppers, mushrooms, garlic and onion. Stir gently, and cook until tender. Add green onions and bean sprouts, stir and cook for a minute. Combine broth and cornstarch in a separate bowl and add the mushroom mixture. Add honey, soy sauce, hoisin sauce, curry powder, cayenne pepper, and ginger. Stir and cook until thickened and bubbly.

3. Add the spaghetti cooked above, and toss.

4. Serve instantly.

Recipe 27

Green Potato Soup

(Ready in 45 minutes with 10 minutes preparation time- serves 4)

Ingredients

- 5 cups chicken broth

- 2 pounds potatoes, peeled and cubed

- 1 pound hot Italian sausage, cubed

- 2 teaspoon pepper

- ½ cup organic milk cream

- 1 pound shredded fresh spinach

- 1/8 teaspoon pepper

Cooking directions

1. Bring ½ of broth and potatoes to boil. Reduce heat, cover and simmer for about 20 minutes. Cook until the potatoes are tender. Mash the cooked potatoes.

2. While potatoes are cooking, fry-drain sausages on paper towels.

3. Add the reaming broth on the mash potatoes, heat and bring to boil. Add greens, cook for about 5 minutes or until wilted. Add pepper, sausage, cream, and salt. Stir gently.

4. Heat and serve.

Slow Cooker Beef Stew

(Ready in 6 hours 20 minutes with preparation time of 20 minutes- serves 4)

Ingredients

- 4 sliced carrots

- 2 ponds cubed beef stew meat

- 1½ cup beef broth

- 1 chopped celery stalk

- 3 diced potatoes

- 1 bay leaf

- 1 minced clove garlic

- 1 chopped onion

- ½ teaspoon salt

- ¼ cup all-purpose flour

- ½ teaspoon black pepper, grounded

- 1 teaspoon of Worcestershire

- 1 teaspoon paprika

Cooking directions

1. In a slower cooker, place meat.

2. Mix salt, pepper and flour, and pour the mixture over meat. Coat the meat with flour mixture, stir. Add bay leaf, onion, garlic, Worcestershire, paprika, carrots, celery, potatoes, and broth. Stir gently.

3. Set the heat to higher, cook for about 6 hours.

4. Ready to serve.

Recipe 29

Maple Apple Chicken Breakfast Sausages

(Ready in 35 minutes with 10 minutes prep time- serves 4)

Ingredients

- 1 pound organic chicken, grounded

- Breakfast sausage seasoning, homemade

- 2 tablespoons maple syrup, organic

- 2 finely grated garlic cloves

- 2 tablespoons of butter

- 4 tablespoons broth

Cooking directions

1. Mix sausage seasoning, ground chicken, maple syrup, grated garlic and diced apple in a large mixing bowl.

2. Shape in to medium sized patties, place onto large plate and set aside.

3. Melt butter in a large pan; fry the patties above until golden brown on both sides for about 15 minutes.

4. Serve four plates.

Recipe 30

Cinnamon Roll Oatmeal

(Ready in 20 minutes with 10 minutes prep time- serves 2)

Ingredients

- ½ cup milk

- ½ cup chicken broth

- 2 cups old fashioned oats, rolled

- 6 tablespoons sugar, powdered

- 1 teaspoon cinnamon

- 2 teaspoon milk

Cooking directions

1. Bring milk and broth to boil in a saucepan

2. Add oats and cinnamon. Lower the heat and heat for 5 minutes or until the oats are tender.

3. Whisk together sugar and 2tsp milk in a small bowl to make icing.

4. Drizzle 2 bowls with icing and serve oatmeal on them. Sprinkle with the remaining cinnamon.

Recipe 31

Braised Pork Pastelon

(Ready in 1 hour 30 minutes with 10 minutes prep time- serves 4)

Ingredients

- 1 cup chicken broth

- 2 pounds cubed pork shoulder

- 1 tablespoon olive oil

- 4 bay leaves

- 1 cup of onion, chopped

- 1 tablespoon olives, sliced

- 1 tablespoon of capers

- 2 tablespoons cilantro leaves, chopped

- 2 tomatoes without seeds, chopped

- 5 plantains, ripe, peeled and sliced

- 2 cups cheddar cheese, shredded

- Black pepper and salt to taste

- 1 tablespoon garlic, sliced

- ½ cup red pepper, chopped

- ½ cup green pepper, chopped

- 2 tablespoon Goya recaito

- 2 tablespoon Goya safrito

- 1 cup Goya sazon

- 2 tablespoon tomato sauce

Cooking directions

1. Heat olive oil in a saucepan. Add pork and season with pepper and salt. Cook the pork and stir gently until pork turns brown on all sides. Remove from pan and set aside.

2. Use the same saucepan to cook garlic until it turns brown, then add onion and cook for 3 minutes.

3. Add peppers and bay leaves, cook for 3 minutes. Add tomato sauce, sofrito, sazon, and recaito. Stir and cook for 3 minutes.

4. Add pork, broth, capers, olives, tomatoes and cilantro. Regulate the heat to medium low. Cook until the pork is tender, about 1 hour.

5. In a deep pan fryer, fry plantains with olive oil. Cook
    until the plantains turn golden brown. Pound the
    plantains using a mortar and season with salt. Set the
    dough aside.

6. Grease a baking dish with butter. Layer half of the
    plantains on the bottom. Add pork stew as the second
    layer. Sprinkle with ½ cheese. Add with the remaining
    plantains. Cover with the other ½ cheese.

7. At 340 degrees F, Bake the mixture until the cheese
    melts, about 10 minutes.

8. Remove the dish from oven and serve.

Recipe 32

Sweet Potato stuffing

(Ready in 4 hours 30 minutes with 15 minutes prep time- serves 5)

Ingredients

- 2 tablespoons butter

- 2 celery stalks, chopped

- ¼ cup onion, chopped

- 3 cups cubed dry bread

- ¼ teaspoon pepper

- ¼ teaspoon rubbed sage

- 1 medium peeled, cubed and cooked sweet potato

- 1/8 cup pecans, chopped

- ½ cup chicken broth

- ¼ teaspoon of poultry seasoning

- Salt to taste

Cooking directions

1. Heat butter in a 6 quart saucepan, add onion and celery, sauté until tender.

2. Add broth and seasonings, stir.

3. Add all the remaining ingredients, stir.

4. Grease a 3 quart with butter. Pour the mixture above

5. Cover and cooker on low heat for about 4 hours

6. Serve

Recipe 33

Butternut Squash Risotto
(Ready in 55 minutes with 10 minutes prep time- serves 4)

Ingredients

- 2 pounds, peeled, seeded and minced butternut squash

- 2 tablespoon butter

- Ground pepper and kosher salt to taste

- 2 cups Arborio rice

- 1 cup white wine, dry

- 4 cups chicken broth

- 1 tablespoon fresh sage, chopped. Have some more for garnishing

- ½ cup Parmesan Cheese, grated

Cooking directions

1. Melt butter in a medium saucepan. Add squash. Add pepper and salt to taste. Keep stirring and cook for about 6 minutes until edges soften

2. Add Arborio rice. To coat with mixture above, stir. Add
    white wine and cook for 2 minutes until all liquid has
    evaporated

3.   Heat reduction to medium low. Add I cup broth mixture.
    Stir gently and cook until all liquid is absorbed. Add
    broth, 1 cup at the time, keep stirring until the liquid is
    absorbed before adding more. Cook for about 40
    minutes

4. Add sage, cheese, and season with salt. Stir gently

5. Serve while hot and garnish with more sage and
    cheese

Recipe 34

Green Bean Casserole
(Ready 45 in minutes with 10 minutes prep time- serves 4)

Ingredients

- 2 cups drained fresh style green beans

- 2 tablespoons all-purpose flour

- 2 tablespoon butter

- 1 tablespoon sugar, white

- ½ cup cream, sour

- ½ cup broth

- 2 tablespoons diced onion

- Salt to taste

- 2 cups cheddar cheese, shredded

- 3 tablespoon butter

- ½ cup buttery round crackers, crumbled

Cooking directions

1. Preheat oven to 175 degrees C

2. In a large skillet 2 tablespoon melt butter over medium heat. Add flour, stir to smoothen and cook for a minute. Add onion, sugar, salt, cream and broth. Add green beans, to coat them stir gently.

3. Pour the mixture into a baking dish. Sprinkle ½ the cheese. In a small bowl, combine remaining butter with cracker crumbs. Add to the dish mixture. Cover with the remaining cheese.

4. Bake until the cheese is bubbly and the top golden brown for about 30 minutes.

5. Ready to serve

Recipe 35

Tomato-less Marinara Sauce

(Ready in 45 minutes with 10 minutes prep time- serves 4)

Ingredients

- 1 tablespoon coconut oil

- 4 minced garlic gloves

- 2 chopped yellow onions

- 1 pound chopped carrots

- 1 medium chopped beet

- Sea salt to taste

- 2 tablespoon lemon juice, fresh

- 1 cup vegetable broth

Cooking directions

1. In a large pan melt oil over medium heat. Add onions and sauté for about 10 minutes or until they are tender and golden brown. Add beet, carrots and broth. Heat to boil. Reduce heat and cook for about 30 minutes until the beets and carrots are tender.

2. Pour the mixture to a blender. Add lemon juice and salt.
    Blend until the mixture is smooth.

3. Serve warm with pasta

Recipe 36

Vegan Creamy Pumpkin Tomato Soup

(Ready in 25 minutes with 10 minutes prep time- serves 4)

Ingredients

- 11/2 cups mushroom broth

- 1 teaspoon olive oil, extra virgin

- ½ chopped yellow onion

- 1 cup strained tomato

- 1 minced clove garlic

- 1 cup of pumpkin puree

- 1 tablespoon of maple syrup

- Salt to taste

- ½ teaspoon cinnamon

- 1 teaspoon minced sage, fresh. Have more

- ½ cup coconut milk

- 1 teaspoon lemon juice, fresh

Cooking directions

1. In a large pot, heat oil. Add onion and sauté for about 8 minutes or until tender. Add garlic and sauté for a minute or until fragrant.

2. Pour the onion mixture to a blender. Add pumpkin, tomato, broth. Cinnamon. Sage, maple and salt. Blend until smooth completely. Pour the soup to the pot and boil it. While at the boiling point, lower the heat. Add milk and lemon juice, stir. Season with salt.

3. Serve warm

Recipe 37

Lentil, Kale and Quinoa Stew

(Ready in 45 minutes with 10 minutes prep time- serves 4)

Ingredients

- 3 chopped celery stalks

- 5 cups vegetable broth

- 1 chopped yellow onion

- 1 tablespoon olive oil

- ½ cup quinoa, dry

- 4 Minced garlic cloves

- ½ teaspoon ginger, grounded

- 11/2 teaspoon cumin, grounded

- ½ teaspoon turmeric, grounded

- Seasoning salt

- 11`/2 cup tomatoes, chopped

- 1 cup red lentils

- 2 cups chopped and tough removed kale

Cooking directions

1. In a large pot melt oil over medium heat. Add onions, celery and carrots. Sauté for 8 minutes or until tender.

2. Add garlic and sauté for minute

3. Add ginger, salt, cumin, turmeric, quinoa, broth and tomatoes. Heat to boil. As the soup boils, reduce the heat. Simmer for 20 minutes or until lentils are tender and vegetables are tender.

4. Add kale, stir and cook until the kale is wilted. Season with salt.

5. Serve warm

Recipe 38

Dairy-Free Corn Chowder
(Ready in minutes 45 with minutes prep time 15- serves 4)

Ingredients

- 4 cups of vegetable broth

- 1 tablespoon olive oil

- 1 chopped red bell pepper

- 1 chopped yellow onion

- 1 pound peeled and cubed Yukon gold potatoes

- 1 teaspoon thyme, dried

- 1 pound organic corn kernels, frozen

- Sea salt and black pepper to taste

- Chives, chopped

Cooking directions

1. In a large pot melt oil. Add onion and pepper, sauté for
   8 minutes or until tender. Add broth, corn potatoes,
   thyme and season with salt. Bring broth to boil. Cover

with a lid and reduce heat. Simmer for 25 minutes or
until the potatoes are tender.

2. Using an immersion blender, blend the mixture directly
in the pot. Leave it to your desired texture.

3. Serve with chopped chives

Recipe 39

Boiled Lobster Tails
(Ready in 25 minutes with 10 prep time - serve 2)

Ingredients

- 2 lobster tails

- Sea salt to taste

- 6 cups of fish broth

- 1 tablespoon melted butter

Cooking directions

1. In a large pan boil the broth

2. Through each lobster tail run a wooden skewer to straighten them.

3. Add salt to taste to the boiling broth

4. Add lobster, reduce heat. Simmer for 8 minutes.

5. Remove from heat and drain excess broth

6. Serve with melted butter

Recipe 40

Thai style Halibut with Coconut Curry Broth

(Ready in27 minutes with 10 prep minutes- serve 4)

Ingredients

- 3/4 cup finely chopped shallots

- 2 teaspoon coconut oil

- 2 teaspoon curry powder

- 2 cups chicken broth

- 1/2 cup coconut milk

- Salt to taste

- 4 skin removed halibut fillet

- 5 spinach leaflets, chopped and steamed

- 1/2 cup fresh cilantro leaves, coarsely chopped

- 2 thinly sliced scallions, green part only

- 2 tablespoon lemon juice, fresh

- Black pepper, grounded

- 2 cups brown rice, cooked

Cooking directions

1. Heat oil in a large saucepan over medium heat. Add shallots, stir and Cook for 5 minutes or until turns brown

2. Add curry paste, stir and cook for about 30 seconds or until fragrant.

3. Add broth, salt and milk. Simmer for 5 minutes or until reduced to 2 cups

4. Season the halibut with salt, about 1/4 teaspoon salt. Layer the fish in the pan and toss gently to coat it with sauce. Cook for about minutes or until the fish flakes easily with a fork.

5. 5 in the bottom of 4 soup plates arrange a layer of steamed spinach. Add fish fillets. Add cilantro, lemon juice, scallions into the sauce, season with pepper and salt. Lay the sauce over the fillets.

6. Serve with rice

Easy Tuna casserole
(Ready in 45 minutes with 10 prep minute)

Ingredients

- 2 cups chicken broth

- 5 ounces drained tuna

- 3 cups macaroni, cooked

- 1 cup Cheddar cheese, shredded

- 11/2 cups of French fried onions

Cooking directions

1. Preheat oven to 275° C

2. Grease a baking dish with butter. Mix tuna, broth and macaroni in it. Cover with cheese.

3. Bake until bubbly, about 25 minutes. Top with fried onions and bake for about 5 minutes.

4. Serve hot

Recipe 42

Traditional Osso Buco
(Ready in 2 hours with 15 minutes prep time-serve 4)

Ingredients

- 2 tablespoon butter

- 1/4 cup all-purpose flour

- 2 pounds cubed veal shanks

- 2 crushes clove garlic

- 1 large chopped carrot

- 1 large chopped onion

- 2/3 cup white wine, dry

- 1 can tomatoes, diced

- 2/3 cup beef stock

- 1/2 cup beef broth

- Pepper and salt to taste

- Gremolata:

    1. 1 minced clove garlic

2. 1/2 cup fresh flat leaf parsley

3. 2 teaspoon lemon Zest, grated

Cooking directions

1. In a small bowl dust the shanks with flour. In a large skillet melt butter over medium heat. Add dusted veal, Cook until turns brown on the outside. Remove from skillet and set aside.

2. In the same skillet, add onion and crushed garlic. Stir and Cook until tender. Add cooked veal. Mix with wine, broth and carrot. Reduce heat and simmer for about 10 minutes.

3. Add beef and tomatoes. Add salt to taste. Reduce heat and simmer for about 11/2 hours or until the meat is tender.

4. Mix lemon zest, minced garlic and parsley in a small bowl to make gremolata.

5. Just before serving sprinkle gremolata over veal.

Corn Bread Dressing

(Ready in 1 hour 15 minutes with 30 minutes prep time- serve 3)

Ingredients

- 1 package corn bread, dry and mix

- 1/4 cup butter

- 2 celery stalks chopped

- 1 chopped small onion

- 2 cups chicken broth

- 2 beaten eggs

- Pepper and salt to taste

- 2 tablespoon sage, dried

Cooking directions

1. Cook corn bread according to the instructions given on the package. Cool and crumble.

2. Preheat oven to 175° C.

3. Grease baking dish with butter

4. Melt butter in a large skillet over medium heat. Add
    onion and celery. Saute until soft.

5. Mix the sautéed celery with eggs, cooked corn bread,
    sage and broth in a large bowl. Season with pepper
    and salt.

6. Pour in the baking dish. Bake for 30 minute at 175
    degrees C.

Recipe 44

Baked Chicken Breast

(Ready35 minutes with 20 minutes prep time- serve 2)

Ingredients

- 2 chicken breasts, boneless and skinless

- 1/4 teaspoon of garlic salt

- 1/2 cup chicken broth

- 1/4 teaspoon of onion powder

- Black pepper for seasoning

Cooking directions

1. Preheat oven to 360 degrees F.

2. Grease baking dish with cooking spray. Add rinsed, patted and dried chicken breasts. Add garlic salt, onion powderand pepper. Add chicken broth.

3. Bake until the chicken is no longer pink, about 20 minutes.

4. Ready to serve.

Recipe 45

Banana Split Oatmeal
(Ready in 15 minutes with 10 prep minutes time- serves 2)

Ingredients

- 2/3 cup quick-cooking oatmeal

- 1/4 teaspoon salt

- 11/2 chicken broth (very hot)

- 1 cup non-fat frozen yogurt

- 1 banana sliced

Cooking directions

1. Mix together oatmeal and salt in a microwave safe cereal bowl. Add broth and stir.

2. Put the microwave on high power for a minute. Stir the oatmeal mixture.

3. Put it on high power again for minute. Stir oatmeal mixture.

4. Put microwave on high power again until the cereal reaches the thickness you want, about 30-60 seconds.

5. Serve with banana slices and frozen yogurt

Conclusion

I hope that by now you have an idea that bone broth is not just about soups as some people have come to think. You can use your homemade broth as a base for different types of healthy meals that come with various health benefits.

As we noted in the introduction, bone broth comes with a number of great benefits. It is generally favored for its anti-inflammatory properties which are contained in the proteins found in bone broth. Before we go, let's just remind you that the way you make your bone broth at home is important to how it tastes. Good cooks will tell you that a badly made broth will taste just as badly as a bowl full of bones.

There are a few things that you should avoid if you want your bone broth to come out well. Remember to clean your bones before you start cooking them. Also, remember to roast the bones. Doing this caramelizes the bines and improves the flavor. If you use an oven you can crank it all the way to 450 degrees F and take all the caramelized stuff remaining on the pan and throw it into the pot when you cook. Do not add to much stuff to the bones. Always ensure that you simmer for long enough and warrant that the broth cools quickly once taken off the stove so that it does not become a breeding ground for bad bacteria.

A good cook is one who is creative in the kitchen. So feel free to play around with the recipes and see if you can come up with new dishes. Remember all the time to keep your ingredients healthy. Where you can prepare or grow your own, by all means do that. Otherwise, enjoy your meal.

Thank you